WALL PILATES

WORKOUT

FOR MEN OVER 50

A Comprehensive Guide to reclaim your health and Strengthening Your Core to boost vitality, Flexibility and Improve Posture.

MARTINE J. TOLEDO

TABLE OF CONTENT

INTRODUCTION

Joe had always been an active man, but as he reached his 50s, he began to experience a decline in his health. Simple tasks that once seemed effortless now left him feeling exhausted and frustrated. His joints ached, his muscles felt weak, and his energy levels plummeted. It seemed like his vitality was slipping away, and he didn't know how to regain it.

One day, while browsing through a local bookstore, Joe stumbled upon a book titled "Wall Pilates Workout for Men over 50." Intrigued, he picked it up and started reading. The book promised a transformative approach to fitness specifically tailored to men like him who were facing the challenges of aging.

As Joe delved into the pages, he discovered a world of exercises, techniques, and guidance that spoke directly to his needs. The author explained how Wall Pilates could not only improve strength and flexibility but also enhance overall health and well-being. Joe felt a flicker of hope ignite within him.

Eager to put the principles into practice, Joe cleared a space in his home and followed the instructions carefully. He aligned his body against the wall, engaging his core and focusing on his breath. The movements were gentle yet effective; targeting muscles he didn't even know he had.

Days turned into weeks, and Joe faithfully continued his Wall Pilates routine. Slowly but surely, he began to notice a change. His joints felt more supple, and his muscles regained their strength. He could reach farther, bend deeper, and stand taller. The constant fatigue he once battled started to fade, replaced by newfound energy and vitality.

Not only did Joe's physical health improve, but he also experienced a positive shift in his mental and emotional well-being. The mindfulness and focus required during his workouts spilled over into other aspects of his life. He felt more centered, more confident, and more capable of facing life's challenges.

Joe's journey with Wall Pilates became a testament to the transformative power of movement and exercise. His friends and family noticed the positive changes in him and were inspired to follow suit. Together, they formed a supportive community, encouraging and motivating one another to embrace a healthier, more active lifestyle.

From a place of uncertainty and declining health, Joe had discovered a path to reclaiming his vitality. Through the simple yet powerful practice of Wall Pilates, he not only regained control over his body but also rediscovered the joy and fulfillment that comes from taking care of oneself. Joe's story serves as a reminder that it's never too late to embark on a journey of self-improvement, and that sometimes, the key to a brighter future lies within the pages of a book.

EXERCISE

General Guidelines

Warm-up:

> - Start by standing with your back against the wall, feet hip-width apart.
> - Gently roll your shoulders back and down.
> - Take a few deep breaths, focusing on relaxing your body.

Wall Squats:

> - Lean against the wall with your feet shoulder-width apart.
> - Slowly lower your body into a squat position, keeping your back against the wall.
> - Hold the squat for a few seconds, then push through your heels to return to the starting position.
> - Repeat for 10-12 repetitions.

Wall Push-Ups:

➢ Stand facing the wall, arms extended, and hands placed shoulder-width apart on the wall.

➢ Lean towards the wall, bending your elbows to perform a push-up motion.

➢ Push back to the starting position.

➢ Repeat for 10-12 repetitions.

Wall Plank:

➢ Place your hands on the wall, shoulder-width apart, and step back until your body is in a straight line.

➢ Engage your core and hold the position for 30 seconds to 1 minute.

➢ Rest and repeat for 2-3 sets.

Wall Leg Raises:

➢ Stand facing the wall, with your hands resting against it for support.

➢ Lift one leg straight out in front of you, keeping it parallel to the floor.

- ➢ Hold for a few seconds, and then lower the leg back down.
- ➢ Repeat with the other leg.
- ➢ Aim for 10-12 repetitions per leg.

Wall Calf Raises:

- ➢ Stand with your toes on an elevated surface, such as a step or sturdy block, and your heels hanging off the edge.
- ➢ Use the wall for balance, and slowly raise your heels as high as possible.
- ➢ Lower your heels back down.
- ➢ Repeat for 10-12 repetitions.

Cool-down:

- ➢ Finish the workout with a few minutes of gentle stretching, focusing on the major muscle groups worked during the session.
- ➢ Take deep breaths and relax your body and mind.

Wall Bridge:

- ➤ Lie on your back with your feet flat against the wall, knees bent.
- ➤ Press your feet into the wall, engaging your gluts and lifting your hips off the ground.
- ➤ Hold for a few seconds, then lower your hips back down.
- ➤ Repeat for 10-12 repetitions.

Wall Shoulder Press:

- ➤ Stand facing the wall with your feet hip-width apart.
- ➤ Place your hands on the wall slightly wider than shoulder-width apart.
- ➤ Bend your elbows and lower your chest towards the wall, keeping your body straight.
- ➤ Push back to the starting position.
- ➤ Repeat for 10-12 repetitions.

Wall Twist:

> ➢ Stand with your back against the wall, feet hip-width apart.
>
> ➢ Extend your arms straight out in front of you, parallel to the floor.
>
> ➢ Slowly rotate your torso to one side, keeping your hips and feet still.
>
> ➢ Return to the center and repeat on the other side.
>
> ➢ Aim for 10-12 repetitions per side.

Wall Side Leg Lifts:

> ➢ Stand sideways with your side against the wall, using your hand for support.
>
> ➢ Lift your top leg out to the side, keeping it straight and parallel to the floor.
>
> ➢ Hold for a few seconds, then lower the leg back down.
>
> ➢ Repeat for 10-12 repetitions per leg.

Wall Hamstring Stretch:

- ➤ Lie on your back with your hips close to the wall.
- ➤ Extend one leg up the wall, keeping it as straight as possible.
- ➤ Feel the stretch in the back of your leg.
- ➤ Hold for 30 seconds to 1 minute, then switch legs and repeat.

Benefit of wall Pilates workout for men over 50

Improved Posture:

Wall Pilate's exercises can help strengthen the muscles responsible for maintaining good posture, such as the core, back, and shoulder muscles. By correcting muscular imbalances and promoting proper alignment, wall Pilates can help men over 50 maintain an upright posture and reduce the risk of postural issues associated with aging.

Increased Strength and Muscle Tone:

As men age, muscle mass tends to decline. Wall Pilates workouts incorporate resistance and bodyweight exercises that target multiple muscle groups simultaneously, helping to build strength and increase muscle tone. This can improve overall functional fitness, making daily activities easier and reducing the risk of age-related muscle weakness.

Enhanced Flexibility and Range of Motion:

Wall Pilates exercises emphasize controlled movements and stretching, which can enhance flexibility and improve joint mobility. This is particularly beneficial for men over 50 who may be experiencing stiffness or reduced range of motion due to age or inactivity.

Core Stability and Balance:

Wall Pilates workouts engage the core muscles, including the abdominal and back muscles, which are essential for stability and balance. By strengthening the core, men over 50 can enhance their balance, coordination, and overall stability, reducing the risk of falls and injuries.

Stress Relief and Mind-Body Connection:

Pilates, including wall Pilates, incorporates mindful breathing and focused movement, promoting relaxation and reducing stress. Engaging in regular wall Pilates workouts can help men over 50 experience improved mental well-being, increased body awareness, and a greater sense of overall calm.

It's important for men over 50 to consult with a qualified Pilates instructor or healthcare professional before starting any new exercise program. They can provide guidance on proper technique, modifications, and ensure that the exercises are appropriate for individual needs and any underlying health conditions.

CHAPTER 1

Wall Roll Down:

Introduction: The Wall Roll Down is a spine-stretching exercise that helps improve flexibility, posture, and core stability.

Instructions:

- Stand with your back against the wall, feet hip-width apart, and the pelvis and spine in neutral alignment.
- Slowly roll down through the spine, articulating one vertebra at a time, keeping the back in contact with the wall.
- Engage the core and roll back up to the starting position, maintaining control throughout the movement.

Benefits:

> ➢ This exercise stretches the spine, strengthens the core, improves posture, and enhances body awareness.

Sets and Repetitions: Start with 2 sets of 8-10 repetitions.

CHATPER 2

Wall Squats:

Introduction: Wall Squats are a lower body strengthening exercise that targets the quadriceps, gluts, and hamstrings.

Instructions:

- ➢ Stand with your back against the wall and feet shoulder-width apart.
- ➢ Slide down the wall into a squat position, keeping your knees aligned with your toes and your back against the wall.
- ➢ Pause for a moment, then push through your heels to return to the starting position.

Benefits:

Wall Squats help improve leg strength, enhance lower body stability, and promote better functional movement.

Sets and Repetitions: Begin with 2 sets of 10-12 repetitions.

CHAPTER 3

Wall Push-Ups:

Introduction: Wall Push-Ups are an upper body strengthening exercise that targets the chest, shoulders, and triceps.

Instructions:

> Stand facing the wall with your arms extended and hands placed on the wall at shoulder height.

> Lean forward, bending your elbows, and lower your chest towards the wall.

> Push back to the starting position by straightening your arms.

Benefits:

Wall Push-Ups improve upper body strength, promote better posture, and enhance pushing movements in daily activities.

Sets and Repetitions: Start with 2 sets of 8-10 repetitions.

CHAPTER 4

Wall Plank:

Introduction: The Wall Plank is a core-strengthening exercise that targets the abdominals, back, and shoulder muscles.

Instructions:

- Stand facing the wall and place your hands on the wall at shoulder height.
- Walk your feet back, maintaining a straight line from your head to your heels, and engage your core.
- Hold the position for a specific duration, focusing on maintaining proper alignment and breathing.

Benefits:

Wall Plank strengthens the core, improves stability, enhances shoulder strength, and promotes better posture.

Sets and Repetitions: Aim for 2 sets, holding the position for 20-30 seconds initially and gradually increasing the duration.

CHAPTER 5

Wall Calf Raises:

Introduction: Wall Calf Raises target the calf muscles and help improve lower leg strength and stability.

Instructions:

- ➢ Stand facing the wall and place your hands on the wall for support.
- ➢ Rise up onto the balls of your feet, lifting your heels as high as possible.
- ➢ Lower your heels back down to the floor.

Benefits:

Wall Calf Raises strengthen the calf muscles, improve ankle stability, and assist in activities like walking and climbing stairs.

Sets and Repetitions: Start with 2 sets of 12-15 repetitions.

CHAPTER 6

Wall Bridge:

Introduction: The Wall Bridge exercise targets the gluts, hamstrings, and core muscles, promoting lower body strength and stability.

Instructions:

> ➢ Lie on your back with your feet flat against the wall and knees bent.
>
> ➢ Engage your core, press your feet into the wall, and lift your hips off the floor, creating a straight line from your knees to your shoulders.
>
> ➢ Pause at the top, then slowly lower your hips back down.

Benefits:

Wall Bridge strengthens the gluts and hamstrings, improves hip stability, and enhances overall lower body strength.

Sets and Repetitions: Begin with 2 sets of 10-12 repetitions.

CHAPTER 7

Wall Rotation:

Introduction: Wall Rotation exercise helps improve spinal mobility, core stability, and rotational strength.

Instructions:

- ➤ Stand with your side facing the wall and place both hands on the wall at shoulder height.
- ➤ Keeping your feet planted, rotate your torso away from the wall as far as comfortable, then rotate back to the starting position.
- ➤ Repeat the movement on the other side.

Benefits:

Wall Rotation increases spine mobility, strengthens the oblique muscles, and enhances rotational movement patterns.

Sets and Repetitions: Aim for 2 sets of 8-10 repetitions on each side.

CHAPTER 8

Wall Side Leg Lifts:

Introduction: Wall Side Leg Lifts target the hip abductor muscles, promoting hip stability and strengthening the outer thighs.

Instructions:

- ➤ Stand sideways to the wall with one hand lightly resting on it for support.
- ➤ Lift the leg farthest from the wall out to the side, keeping the leg straight or slightly bent.
- ➤ Lower the leg back down with control.

Benefits:

Wall Side Leg Lifts strengthen the hip abductors, improve hip stability, and assist in maintaining balance.

Sets and Repetitions: Start with 2 sets of 10-12 repetitions on each leg.

CHAPTER 9

Introduction: The Wall Shoulder Stretch helps improve shoulder mobility, release tension, and promote better posture.

Instructions:

> ➢ Stand facing the wall and place your forearm against the wall at shoulder height.
> ➢ Slowly rotate your body away from the wall, feeling a stretch in the front of your shoulder and chest.
> ➢ Hold the stretch for a specific duration, then switch sides.

Benefits:

Wall Shoulder Stretch increases shoulder mobility, releases tightness, and helps alleviate upper body tension.

Sets and Repetitions: Hold the stretch for 20-30 seconds on each side, repeating 2-3 times.

CHAPTER 10

Wall Abdominal Crunches:

Introduction: Wall Abdominal Crunches engage the core muscles, specifically the rectus abdominals, to strengthen the abdominal region.

Instructions:

- ➢ Sit on the floor with your back against the wall and your knees bent.
- ➢ Cross your arms over your chest, engage your core, and lift your upper body off the floor, curling towards your knees.
- ➢ Lower yourself back down with control.

Benefits:

Wall Abdominal Crunches strengthen the core, improve abdominal muscle tone, and support better posture.

Sets and Repetitions: Begin with 2 sets of 12-15 repetitions.

As always, it's important to consult with a qualified Pilates instructor or healthcare professional before attempting these exercises, particularly if you have any underlying health conditions.

CHAPTER 11

Wall Hamstring Stretch:

Introduction: The Wall Hamstring Stretch targets the hamstrings, promoting flexibility and reducing tightness in the back of the thighs.

Instructions:

> ➤ Lie on your back with your hips close to the wall and legs extended against the wall.
>
> ➤ Flex one foot and raise that leg up towards the ceiling, keeping the other leg resting against the wall.
>
> ➤ Hold the stretch for a specific duration, feeling the stretch in the back of the elevated leg, then switch sides.

Benefits:

Wall Hamstring Stretch increases hamstring flexibility, improves lower body mobility, and aids in relieving tightness. Sets and Repetitions: Hold the stretch for 20-30 seconds on each side, repeating 2-3 times.

CHAPTER 12

Wall Triceps Dips:

Introduction: Wall Triceps Dips target the triceps, promoting upper body strength and toning the back of the arms.

Instructions:

> ➤ Stand facing away from the wall and place your hands on the wall, shoulder-width apart, fingers pointing downwards.
> ➤ Walk your feet forward, creating an angle with your body, and position your feet hip-width apart.
> ➤ Bend your elbows and lower your body towards the wall, then push back up to the starting position.

Benefits:

Wall Triceps Dips strengthen the triceps, improve upper body pushing strength, and enhance arm definition.

Sets and Repetitions: Start with 2 sets of 8-10 repetitions.

CHAPTER 13

Wall Hip Flexor Stretch:

Introduction: The Wall Hip Flexor Stretch targets the hip flexor muscles, improving hip flexibility and reducing tightness.

Instructions:

- ➢ Kneel on one knee with your back against the wall and the other foot positioned in front of you.
- ➢ Gently press your hips forward, feeling a stretch in the front of the kneeling leg.
- ➢ Hold the stretch for a specific duration, then switch legs.

Benefits:

Wall Hip Flexor Stretch increases hip flexor flexibility, improves hip mobility, and helps alleviate tightness.

Sets and Repetitions: Hold the stretch for 20-30 seconds on each leg, repeating 2-3 times.

CHAPTER 14

Wall Side Plank:

Introduction: The Wall Side Plank exercise targets the obliques, core muscles, and shoulder stability, promoting overall core strength.

Instructions:

> ➢ Stand sideways to the wall and place your forearm against the wall, elbow directly below your shoulder.
> ➢ Walk your feet away from the wall, extending your legs, and balance on the side of your bottom foot.
> ➢ Hold the side plank position, keeping your body aligned, and engage your core.

Benefits:

Wall Side Plank strengthens the oblique's, improves core stability, and enhances shoulder strength and stability.

Sets and Repetitions: Aim for 2 sets, holding the position for 20-30 seconds on each side.

CHAPTER 15

Wall Lunge:

Introduction: Wall Lunges target the quadriceps, gluts, and hamstrings, promoting lower body strength and toning.

Instructions:

> ➢ Stand facing the wall and place your hands on the wall for support.
> ➢ Take a step back with one foot and lower your body into a lunge position, keeping the front knee aligned with your toes.
> ➢ Push through the front heel to return to the starting position.

Benefits:

Wall Lunges strengthen the lower body, improve leg muscle tone, and enhance lower body stability and balance.

Sets and Repetitions: Start with 2 sets of 10-12 repetitions on each leg.

Remember to listen to your body, maintain proper form, and consult with a qualified Pilates instructor or healthcare professional before attempting these exercises, particularly if you have any underlying health conditions.

CHAPTER 16

Introduction: The Wall Single Leg Balance exercise improves balance, stability, and proprioception.

Instructions:

> - Stand facing the wall and place your hands on the wall for support.
> - Lift one leg off the ground, bending the knee to a comfortable height.
> - Hold the single-leg balance position, focusing on maintaining stability and proper alignment.

Benefits:

Wall Single Leg Balance enhances balance, strengthens the lower body, and improves overall stability.

Sets and Repetitions: Aim for 2 sets of 30-60 seconds on each leg.

CHAPTER 17

Introduction: The Wall Chest Opener exercise stretches the chest muscles, promoting better posture and relieving upper body tension.

Instructions:

- Stand sideways to the wall and place your forearm against the wall at shoulder height.
- Slowly rotate your body away from the wall, feeling a stretch in the chest and front shoulder.
- Hold the stretch for a specific duration, then switch sides.

Benefits:

Wall Chest Opener increases chest mobility, opens up the front of the shoulders, and improves upper body posture.

Sets and Repetitions: Hold the stretch for 20-30 seconds on each side, repeating 2-3 times.

CHAPTER 18

Wall Pike:

Introduction: The Wall Pike exercise targets the core, shoulders, and hip flexors, promoting core strength and shoulder stability.

Instructions:

- ➢ Assume a push-up position with your feet against the wall and hands shoulder-width apart on the ground.
- ➢ Engage your core, lift your hips and walk your feet up the wall, bringing your body into an inverted V shape.
- ➢ Slowly lower your hips back down to the starting position.

Benefits:

Wall Pike strengthens the core, improves shoulder stability, and enhances overall body control and stability.

Sets and Repetitions: Start with 2 sets of 8-10 repetitions.

CHAPTER 19

Introduction: The Wall Reverse Plank exercise targets the gluts, hamstrings, core, and shoulders, promoting full-body strength and stability.

Instructions:

- Sit with your legs extended in front of you, back against the wall, and hands placed on the ground behind you.
- Press through your hands and lift your hips off the ground, creating a straight line from your head to your heels.
- Hold the reverse plank position, engaging your core and squeezing your gluts.

Benefits:

Wall Reverse Plank strengthens the posterior chain, improves core stability, and enhances shoulder and hip mobility.

Sets and Repetitions: Aim for 2 sets, holding the position for 20-30 seconds.

CHAPTER 20

Wall Scissor Kicks:

Introduction: Wall Scissor Kicks target the lower abs, hip flexors, and quadriceps, promoting core strength and lower body stability.

Instructions:

> ➤ Lie on your back with your legs extended against the wall, hands resting by your sides or under your hips for support.
> ➤ Lift one leg off the wall and lower the other leg towards the wall, then switch legs in a scissor-like motion.
> ➤ Continue alternating leg movements while keeping your lower back pressed into the floor.

Benefits;

Wall Scissor Kicks strengthen the lower abs, improve hip flexor strength, and enhance lower body stability.

Sets and Repetitions: Start with 2 sets of 10-12 repetitions on each leg.

CONCLUSION

In conclusion, incorporating wall Pilates exercises into your workout routine can bring immense benefits for men over 50. These exercises specifically target various muscle groups, enhance flexibility, improve balance, and promote overall strength and stability. By utilizing the support of a wall, these exercises provide a safe and effective way to engage the body and reap the rewards of Pilates.

By consistently practicing wall Pilates exercises, you can expect to experience increased core strength, improved posture, enhanced mobility, and reduced muscle tightness. These exercises are designed to cater to the specific needs of men over 50, considering factors such as flexibility, joint health, and muscle tone.

Embracing a fitness routine that includes wall Pilates can have a transformative impact on your overall well-being.

Not only will you notice physical changes, but you will also experience increased confidence, mental clarity, and a sense of accomplishment. Remember, it's never too late to prioritize your health and fitness.

So, why wait? Seize this opportunity to adopt and adapt wall Pilates exercises into your daily life. Make a commitment to yourself, and let the wall be your support system as you embark on this journey. Embrace the challenge, stay consistent, and witness the positive changes unfold in your body and mind. Your health and vitality are worth every effort. Start today and pave the way to a stronger, healthier, and more fulfilling life. You've got this!